Appetite Control System

Ruth Bowyer

For anyone struggling with their weight or overeating.

We have all heard the advice that eating less and exercising more is the only way to lose weight. But this isn't true and just brings feelings of hopelessness. After all, not everyone who is inactive is overweight. But is there a way out of all this? What have we overlooked?

Index

It seems the body does have an appetite control system but that it is a matter of chance as to whether or not, or how much we use it.

Located in the **outer** gums and surrounding areas, the mechanism which can send the message to the brain to make us stop wanting to eat is activated by pressure and friction.

Originally, this would have been automatic and closely associated with the act of eating. Gnawing and working at our food using our teeth and involving outer gums and surrounding outer mouth - particularly the front - and by particular postures and habits. But as we don't gnaw at our food these days, those various habits and postures have to substitute. And in this modern world this can be hit and miss.

It is important to remember that for these controls to work fully, and to be healthy, we have to eat. Hunger and the need to eat what the body requires will override their effect.

This may sound simple but bear with it. When there are two or more 'faults' in a system it is difficult to recognise a problem as another fault uncorrected will obscure the effect of the other(s) being put right.

There are all kinds of ways of contacting and stimulating this appetite off switch, both directly and indirectly. Some of these occur during daily grooming, e.g. brushing teeth and gums, shaving, checking shaved area, cleaning your face and applying make-up (figs 1-4). Any external pressure, assuming it is adequate, is transmitted through your flesh to the outer gums beneath stimulating the mechanism which sends that message to the brain.

We all do these things to a greater or lesser extent and in differing amounts of pressure. Most grooming happens in the morning, which is also when people are more able to resist eating.

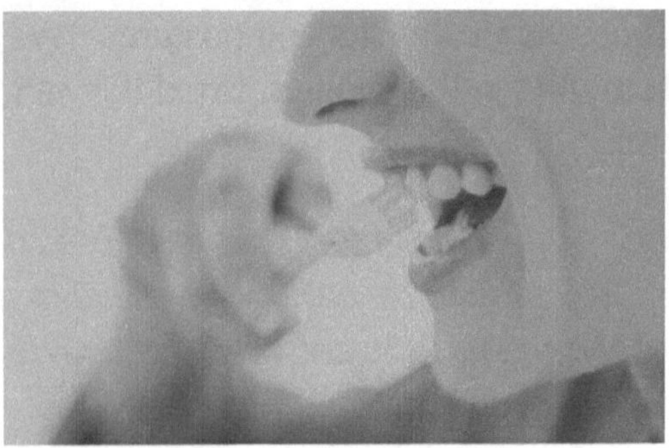

Fig 1

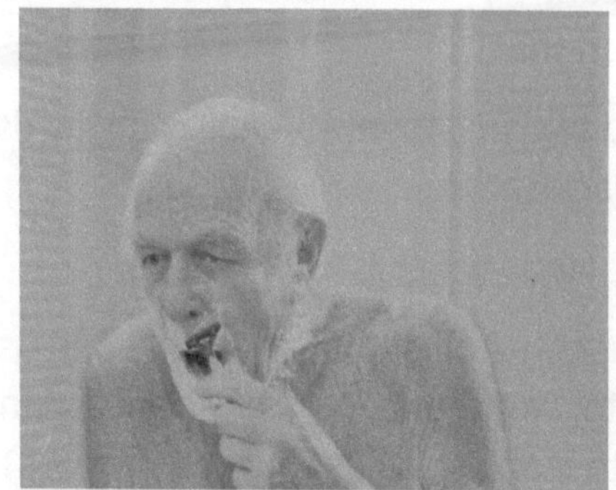

Fig 2

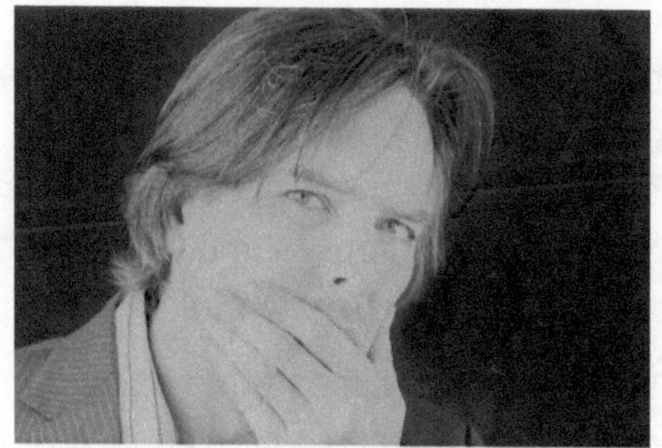

Fig 3

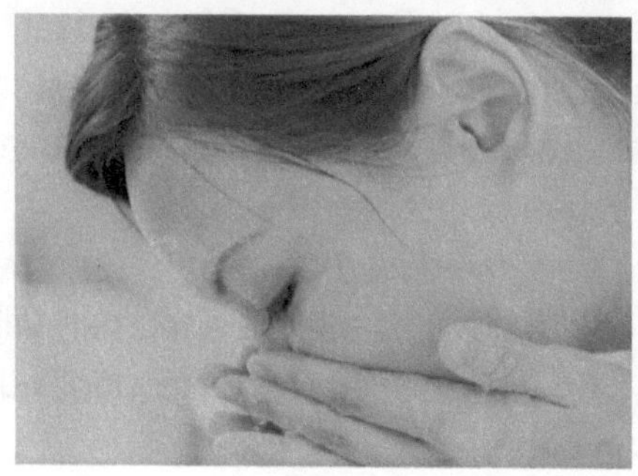

Fig 4

There are other ways too of stimulating the body's appetite controls. For instance, the way we sit is very important.

There are two main ways: leaning forwards, and leaning backwards.

<u>Sitting leaning forwards</u>.

For example, when sitting at a table and using it to read, write, work, play games, socialise, and so on, we tend to lean forwards, put our elbow(s) on the table and support the head with our hand(s) on our mouth (figs 5-8).

We often move our hand position quite a lot when we do this, rubbing the face, leaning on a hand or holding the lower face. All of this results in pressure on the outer mouth, which is transmitted through to the outer gums, stimulating those senses.

Sitting up at a table for meals and leaning forward a little each time you put something in your mouth, also helps (fig 9). This will compress your stomach and help you feel full more quickly. In fact, this can help at any time; bending , doing housework, digging at ground level, exercises, etc. Anything, whether active or not, can help.
If you are very overweight, however, this won't be possible or effective as a large abdomen will prevent it. In which case, more frequent gum stimulation can help.

The easiest way to activate your appetite controls is to rub your upper and lower outer gums quite firmly with a clean cloth on a couple of fingers for about 20 seconds several times a day. Perhaps before a meal. A clean cotton flannel or towel is good. Take care if your gums aren't healthy. Include the frenulum which is the small fold of tissue at the very front between lip and gum.

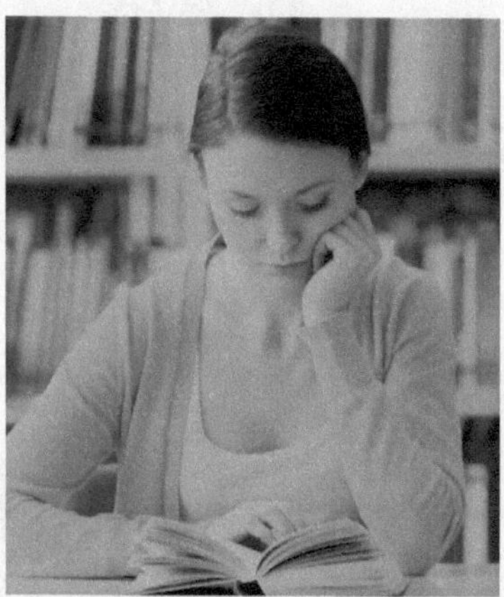

Fig 5

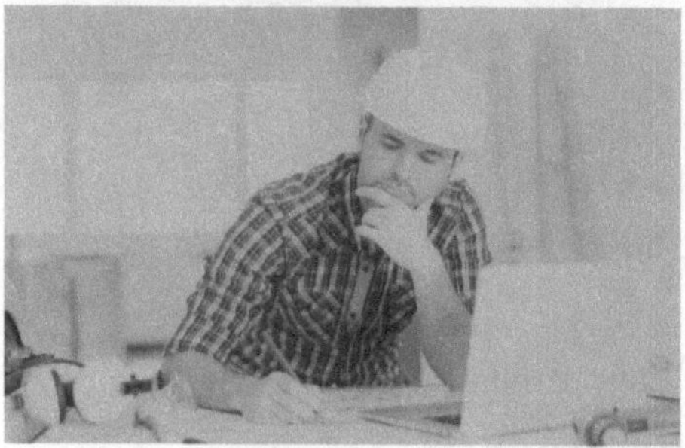

Fig 6

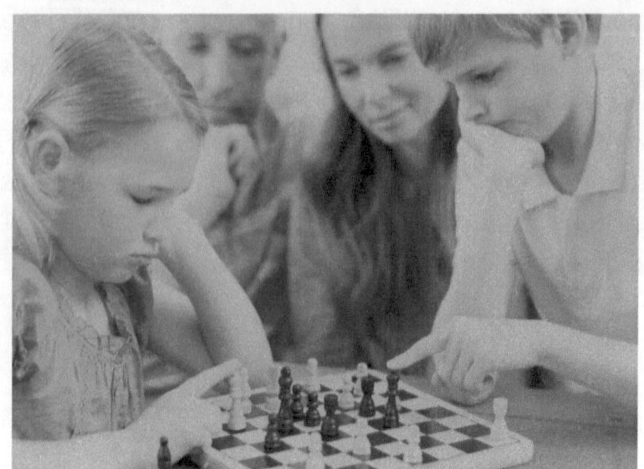

Fig 7

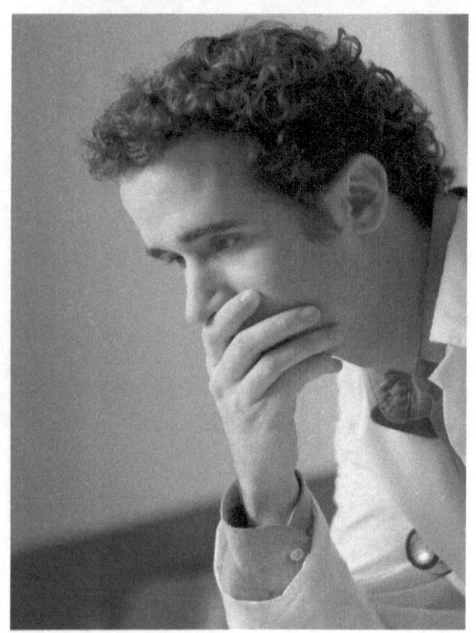

Fig 8

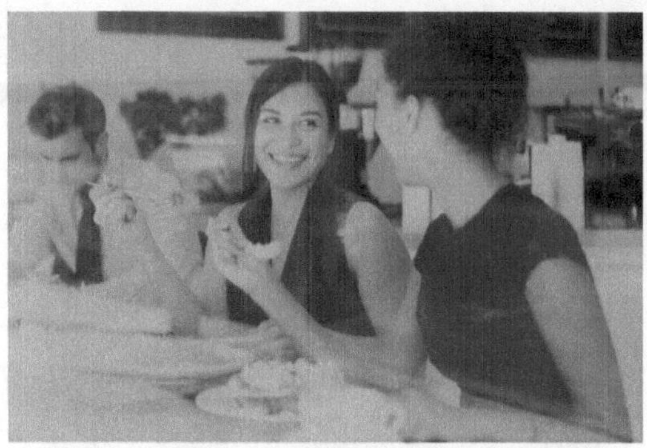

Fig 9

<u>Sitting leaning backwards</u>.

These days in the west we all have soft armchairs, recliners and sofas, and many of us spend a lot of time sitting in them, leaning backwards and supported from behind, very often watching TV (fig 10). While it may be lovely and relaxing, this will not promote pressure on the mouth from hands supporting the head from the front, nor will it produce stomach compression.

In addition, (figs 11 & 12), the 'full' message from natural stomach compression won't activate until you are unnecessarily full, if at all. Add to this an unsatisfactory diet and the perfect storm for overeating is created.

Standing while eating has the same effect. (fig 13)

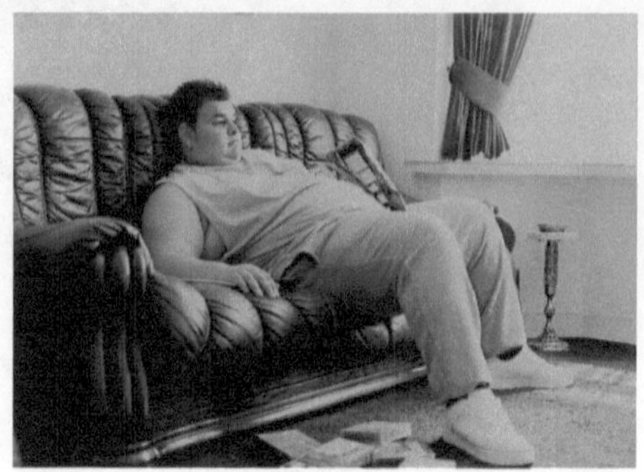

Fig 10

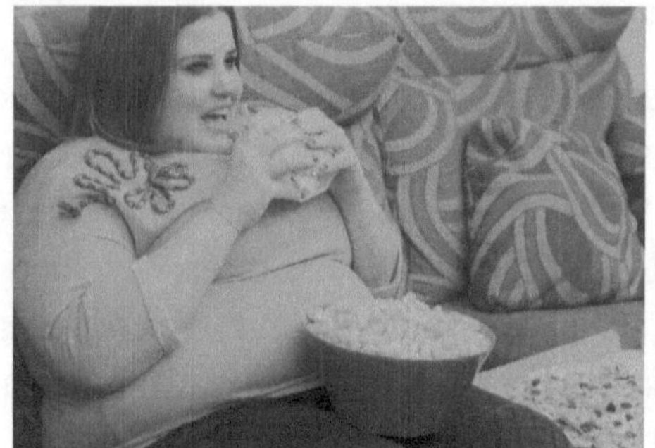

Fig 11

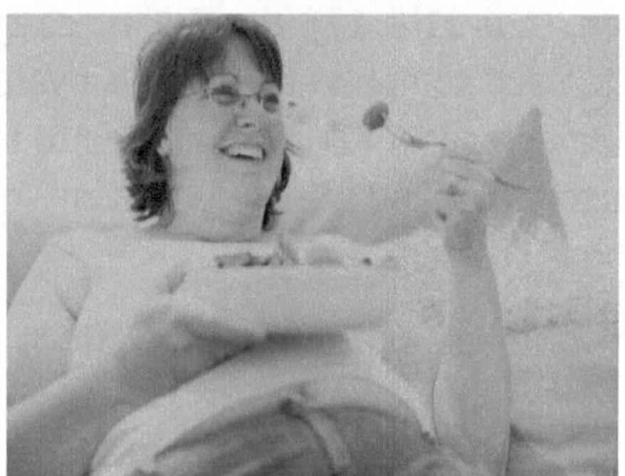

Fig 12

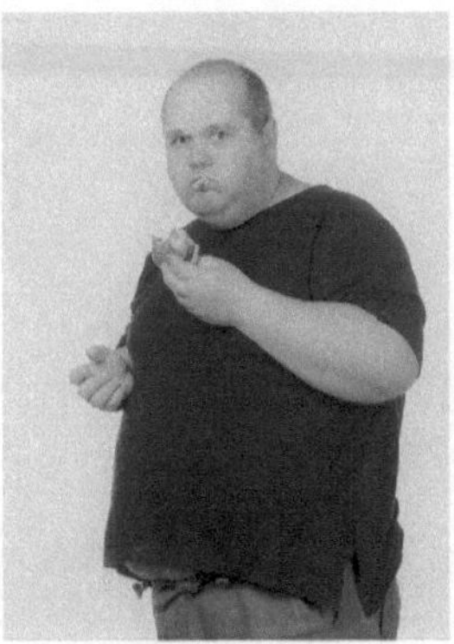

Fig 13

Lying down and sleeping positions.

Being fully at rest, lying down, normally includes various positions. Lying on the side brings helpful contact to the side and front of the mouth from hands or pillow (fig 14). This will provide some pressure to those controls. If you nap take the time to lie on your side.

Even when we sleep or rest on our backs, we don't stay in one position for long periods. Normally, we would move from time to time by rolling over to ease ourselves and this will then include other positions. Large body size, however, can mean that lying on your back or resting leaning backwards is easiest, and can make changing position difficult. Soft modern arm chairs and beds can also make changing position feel unnecessary.

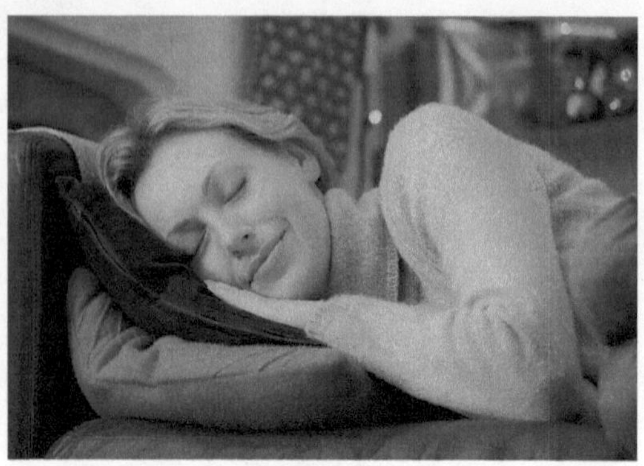

Fig 14

All these easy ways can make the difference between the message to stop eating being sent to/from your brain, or not.

As the mouth and stomach are the parts of the body we use for eating and receiving food, it is logical that they should play a big part in regulating the size of the appetite and stop us wanting to eat before we overeat.

However, to fully satisfy the appetite we have to eat what we need.

The nutritional side.

If you change your habits, or your work changes, or something influences your regular patterns so that you find you are leaning backwards or standing upright more often, or lying on your back, or contacting your face less often, then you can lose some or all of the controls that should be quietly running in the background. You may find that your appetite begins to grow (which may already be your state).

When we put on weight or fear putting on weight, we tend to start all sorts of 'diets', usually low fat ones. But these can make the problem worse, leading to unsatisfying nutritional imbalances, food cravings, and ultimately more weight gain. If you don't eat what you need to satisfy the nutritional part of your appetite then your physical appetite controls (in outer gums) won't work so well.

It's important, therefore, to remember that for appetite controls to work, you have to eat what your body needs. Your good health depends upon you eating good nutrition.

For decades we have been told that low fat is healthy. But is it? It may depend on how we go about it.

Undoubtedly, a diet consisting largely of fats, sugar and starch is not good. All those cakes, biscuits, sweets, chips, crisps, etc., just don't contain the proper nutrition we need to satisfy the appetite and be healthy.

But cutting fats down too much, or out of, our meals — our proper food, containing protein —will just create cravings for fats and those fat/sugar/starch extras. It can also create a preference for them over proper meals.

So *trying* to eat less fat can have the opposite effect at the end of the day or in the long run and make you eat more overall, and in a bad way. And if you don't eat enough fats, particularly with your proper food, your body can go into famine mode, converting other food to body fat, and lowering its basal metabolic rate.

To satisfy the appetite nutritionally and be healthy, we have to eat what we need.

Protein (meat, vegetarian - if complete, fish, dairy, etc.)

Fats (including some types of oil.)

Carbohydrates (vegetables, fruit, whole grains, pulses, but with conditions on starch (see later section). There is much discussion on carbs.

Vitamins and minerals; should be automatically provided if you eat fresh varied food.

We need a certain proportion of what we eat to be fats as they provide satisfaction value in meals and provide the fuel for our bodies to be able to make full use of all the nutrients.

Proportion means relative to how much of everything else you eat. So the more of everything else you eat the more fat/oil you will need. Equally the less of everything else, the less fat/oil needed. Ideally, we need to eat them at the same time as protein and some carbs – maybe vegetables - in meals for our bodies to be able to make full and satisfying use of all the nutrients. Too little relative to everything else and we will continue wanting to eat.

If the fats you do eat are mainly hard fats it may be better to eat more oil instead. There is also much debate about hard fats v. seed oils. Olive oil comes from fruit.

Because we have an abundance of all sorts of things to eat and so can easily overeat, we need to eat our food and fats in the most effective and satisfying way. And it is by eating all food groups together largely as meals that we do this. Meals have worked well for centuries. They are the most efficient way of eating in terms of amounts eaten to satisfy the appetite. This, along with an appetite made smaller by adequate use of your physical appetite controls, is the best way to bring your eating under control.

For many people dieting means trying to eat less fat/oil by cutting them right down in meals. But if you do this your meals will be unsatisfying and you will want to go on eating.

And because fats are so important (and they make food delicious), you will eventually give in and eat them. When you do, you may well choose things such as cakes, biscuits, chips and packet snacks; whatever is to hand.

Then, having eaten them, you may feel guilty and try to balance things by cutting fats out of your next meal. So eating like this creates an unsatisfying imbalance and encourages you to overeat, because the message from your body and brain that you have eaten what you need doesn't get sent at the time of eating.

In effect, you eat your real food and fats at different digestion times.

This way of eating can also create a preference for fat, starch and sugar food items over healthy satisfying meals. You come to think that as you know you are going to eat them anyway, you might as well eat them in the first place and try to save calories by not eating proper meals. But those biscuits, chips, cakes and many processed snacks won't satisfy your appetite properly, particularly if you eat them at the expense of real food. They simply don't contain the necessary nutrition the body needs. You end up eating fats anyway but in an unhealthy way leaving your body unsatisfied nutritionally.

There are all sorts of distortions in the way we can eat when things get out of hand. Had you eaten a satisfying proportion of good fats in healthy meals in the first place, you wouldn't want all those extras. Your body wouldn't be feeling deprived and keep telling you to eat.

Fats become more desirable the more you deny yourself them, because they're nutritionally necessary. They provide much of the fuel our bodies need.

No matter how much we use the control senses in the outer mouth and stomach, we still need to eat what we need to satisfy the nutritional side of the appetite and be healthy.

Eating in time

Having regular, satisfying meals - along with using your appetite controls enough - is the best way to stop yourself from picking at food all the time, particularly if you are at home or near food for a lot of the time.

It is well-documented that a large percentage of overweight people miss breakfast, or don't eat a satisfactory one. As a result, you start each day needing nourishment and if you don't fulfil this need then your appetite will be pushing at you from the start and getting stronger.

This applies to all mealtimes but particularly to breakfast, your <u>first</u> food after your main rest and fast, whatever the time. It's very important. You don't need to eat straight away after getting up. Eating in time tells our bodies that food is available and helps diminish the appetite. It gives us strength and energy for the time ahead.

Breakfast is often the easiest meal to miss as there is likely to be some appetite-control effect from morning grooming and probably from lying on your side or front. So for those trying not to eat, it would be better to eat a good breakfast particularly if you are at home or near food all the time.

When you use your physical appetite controls, you will be able to make decisions about what you eat, rather than just letting your appetite rule you and grabbing whatever is available. Having real, good ingredients and foods available or easily prepared, and eating regular meals so that you're never over-hungry will help. Portion size is important, too.

Once your body has adjusted to having all it needs at each mealtime, and you have a smaller appetite, your body will stop feeling the need to hoard fat.

Improve your metabolic rate

When needs are met regularly and the appetite controls are activated, your body feels secure about its supply of nutrition.

By eating what you need and adjusting your appetite so that it functions effectively, your basal metabolism (that which is used for involuntary processes such as heartbeat, conversion of food, body heat, breathing, brain activity and so on) will work at its optimum rate and use up more energy than it would do otherwise, even if you are sitting still. A fully nourished body will no longer feel the need to conserve energy or convert food to body fat, or hoard body fat for what it feels is the threat of famine brought on by denial dieting, bingeing or a poor diet.

As we don't have a real famine and can continue eating, we shouldn't be threatening our bodies with it by going on imbalanced diets and trying not to eat.

In other words, eating less overall and using up more energy can be further helped by eating what you need in the first place and boosting your basal metabolic rate.

Diet is what we end up eating overall. Low fat 'diets' can make us eat more overall; e.g., 2000 calories from protein and fats will have a different effect on the metabolism than 2000 calories from starch, fats and sugar.

Protein

This provides the building and repair materials for the body. But if the body receives insufficient fuel in the form of fats, or fats and carbs, it will use the protein for fuel in preference to using it for building and repair. No other nutrient can substitute for protein for these purposes, so with inadequate fuel, you reduce your body's ability to heal itself.

Fats (including oils)

Amongst other things, they provide fat soluble vitamins. The use our bodies make of the fats we eat is a different process from using body fat. Denying yourself fats in the hope that your body will use up its reserves of fat doesn't make sense and doesn't work. Cutting them down in real food (meals), only to binge on them later, doesn't give you fat with your proper food at the same digestion time.

Carbohydrates

These include fruit, vegetables, sugar and starch – e.g. flours from grains, (bread, pasta, pastry etc), rice, pulses and starchy vegetables. If you eat a lot of starch then a lower intake may be better. See blood pressure section.

Salt

We need salt. However, mass-produced, processed foods contain large amounts of it. If what you eat is fresh and healthy and your appetite isn't over-large, then the amount of salt you need and find necessary for taste will be modest.

<u>Fibre</u>

When a normal, reasonably varied diet is eaten, the bulk and natural fibre content of grains, pulses, fruit and vegetables helps to pass waste through. However, the fact that some fibre is good doesn't mean that lots of it is better. Excess fibre such as bran can prevent the body from absorbing calcium. In extreme cases it can clog the intestines. Constipation can go hand in hand with low-fat diets. Eating more fat/oil can help relieve this.

In satisfactory proportions, fruit and vegetables provide bulk yet their high water content makes a meal less dense. But eating them in excess instead of a reasonably balanced meal just won't satisfy your appetite for long.

Control aggression and mood swings

There's another drawback to dieting: it affects our mood. Many emotional states become distorted when fundamental nutrition and appetite control are not right.

When we get hungry, our aggression rises. We can get snappy and irritable while waiting to eat, particularly if there is a delay. As with animals living naturally, aggression where there is real competition for food is an aid to survival. When dieting, people are often irritable and intolerant. Continuously trying to avoid what you need and want and struggling not to eat when you want to eat will make you feel aggressive or bad tempered. We have imbalanced diets and low-fat food thrust at us all the time. We also have every kind of food to tempt us when our fuel-starved or confused bodies eventually get the better of us.

The resulting loss of control of the appetite, the malnourishment, binge eating, weight gain, unsatisfactory nutrition, and so on, can lead to negativity, intolerance and depression.

Good nutrition and adequate control support many good aspects of our lives, including our normal chemical balance and, consequently, our emotional balance.

Children

Imposing unsatisfactory nutrition on children, as is now often the case in these days of "dieting", can be the cause of their poor eating habits. When given otherwise good, healthy meals/food, but low fat/oil they find it unpalatable and so refuse it. Bodies and minds unencumbered by all the talk of "dieting" will go by their instinct. If decent food, without much fat, is offered and tasted, their systems won't want it. They'd rather have the chips, cakes, sweets, biscuits, packet snacks, etc. for the fats they instinctively know they need. A body which then doesn't receive healthy, wholesome nutrition, but largely fat, sugar and starchy foods, often full of preserving and flavouring additives, will be affected.

This lack of body-and-brain-building and repairing nutrition causes problems and may show up as behavioural abnormalities in the child, or adult, or at least as stress and an inability to concentrate on anything for long. Having an incomplete or poor diet lowers the body and brain's ability to be at their best.

Equally, a child who has no choice but to eat very low-fuel food, very often in a fad diet, is likely to develop other problems related to poor nutrition and a very strong desire, when independent, for all the tempting easy-grab foodstuff that surrounds us.

The range of foods often eventually preferred by children are the commercial meals aimed at them, plus branded "chips", sugar and fat-filled rubbish, drinks full of saccharine, sugar and additives, sweets, packet snacks etc. By their very presence everywhere, these force many parents into giving their children what they want, which is what all their peers are eating and which, therefore, they assume must be O.K!

Children do childish things if left to their own impulses, which is fine and natural. But there are many exceptions which shouldn't be ignored and which leave room for learning. Nutrition is one of those exceptions. Foodstuff dressed up in boxes, packets, forms and shapes, and coloured drinks, all designed and promoted to attract childish attention, will tend to be eaten at the expense of real, good, healthy nutrition.

How can a child, left to its own choosing, know from all the visual misinformation presented to it, the traditional knowledge and human skills of cooking, and learn the original common sense about good eating, or the down-side of eating a poor-quality diet? They'll go by the outer packing, known from their favourite mass-media characters, or from symbols which make the children feel they are the same as all the others, or are part of a gang, or group.

Those taken in by it don't have the knowledge or normal guidance to do any different or to realise that apparently friendly or strong characters will promote rubbish. This tends to set a pattern for life and the very valuable skills and knowledge about good cooking and nutrition are being lost to many people as a result. And, worse than that, all those foodstuffs promoted by visual misinformation are taking their place.

Exercise

Not everyone who is inactive is overweight.

This is evident from the number of people who don't, or can't exercise and yet who are not overweight. So lack of exercise is not the fundamental issue involved in weight gain. Equally, not all overweight people are inactive. While exercise is good and contributes to effective circulation, overall health and mobility, it is quite possible to remain at a stable and healthy weight without exercising. Though everyone who can exercise should. Normal activities such as housework and gardening can provide plenty. And any exercise at your level of ability is better than none.

Achieve balance

In substance, we are what we eat. What we do with our bodies is also relevant. Good basic health and the ability to heal quickly come largely from eating good food – largely protein and fats - and from allowing our bodies and minds to rest fully. This includes resting from the demands of appetite so our bodies can constantly realign themselves to the best advantage.

Realignment is about bringing our bodies into balance for optimum efficient functioning, good health and a sense of well-being.

A constantly 'on' appetite will get in the way of realignment by keeping our focus on food, which is a distraction from the pursuit of well-being. But the postures and habits that involve putting our hands to our face, applying pressure to those most forward senses and bending the body forwards (figs 15 & 16), not only control the appetite, but also help beneficial realignment right down to the cellular level. They allow the body's ability to relieve pain and heal quickly to come to the fore. In addition, they allow us to concentrate more on things other that the acquisition and eating of food. (fig 17).

The appetite is on until it is turned off

It needs to be this way round, otherwise life wouldn't exist so successfully. There is no life without the appetite leading to nutrition.

It is vital; we need our appetite to remind us to eat because we need to eat to live. Ever since ancient times it has always been important that the appetite was turned off when enough had been eaten. For a species to survive and continue it needed to be fit and healthy, not hindered by an overweight body that might allow it to be caught and end up as prey for other species.

Today we can live unhealthily because we are protected. We don't have to search for our food, escape from predators or rely on our fitness for survival. But just because we can survive and still be eating the wrong foods, and too much food, that doesn't mean it is a good thing. If we are ruled and driven by an unstoppable appetite, then life becomes pretty miserable. Other aspects of ourselves - for instance, our creativity, our ability to think or concentrate, feel content, peaceful, happy - become overwhelmed and lost under the constant craving for food.

We should all have the size of appetite for our individual needs and energy expenditure. The less active you are, the less you need to eat. So being **in**active (resting) should produce a smaller appetite. This can come abut by resting/sitting in ways that **do** stimulate your appetite controls adequately.

What we need is to put the appetite in its place, to have it let us know when we need to eat, and switch off when we have eaten enough. Then we need to be able to forget about food and get on with living until it is necessary for us to eat again. The good feelings and normal physical and mental energy resulting from the natural, satisfied, fully-rested and well-nourished state help to bring about a positive state of body and mind that we should all enjoy as a matter of course.

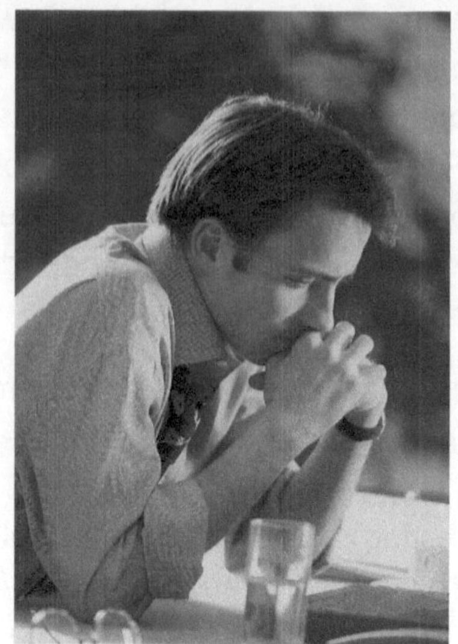

Fig 15

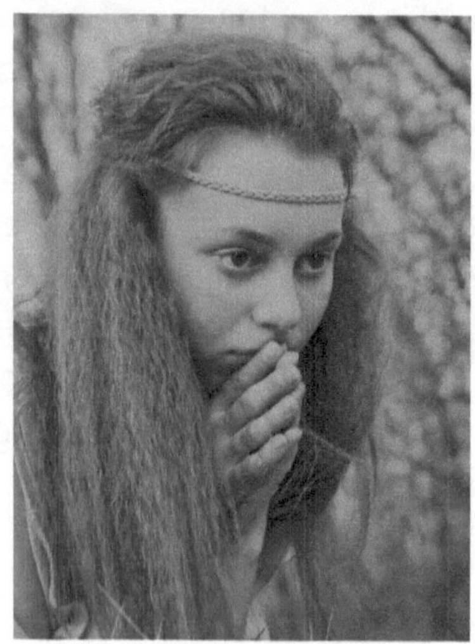

Fig 16

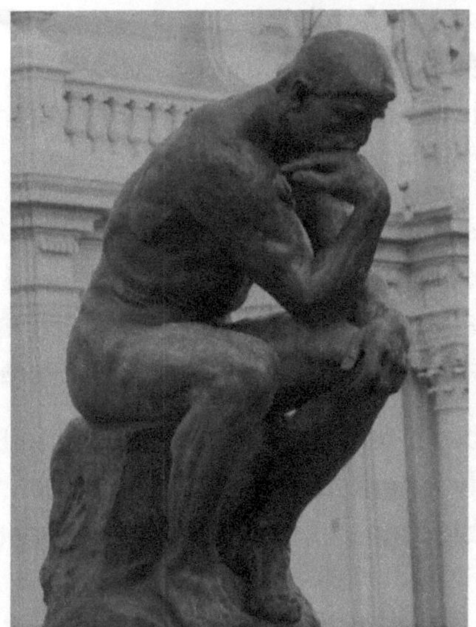

Fig 17

Blood pressure

Despite having found how to control my appetite, my blood pressure has remained persistently high. But lately I have been experimenting with my food and have found how to reduce it a lot.

This is a record of my experiences and findings. My explanation as to why it works may be completely wrong, but it works for me.

Broadly, just from the food point of view, I think it is to do with proportion of protein and fats to **certain** forms of carbohydrate/starch, and how to include some of those carbs/starch in a beneficial way.

I have a strong family history of strokes. My father had one at 80 and died three days later. My mother at 69 and was badly disabled for the rest of her life. She died aged 92.

I don't want to take medication for BP and have tried to deal with it by food and lifestyle. I don't smoke, have occasional alcoholic drinks, am fairly active and had been on low salt for several years.

I do wonder if tendency to essential high BP is more likely inherited eating habits, or eating unavoidable ingredients, rather than genetic.

Although my BP was usually high — in the range of 160-200 sys 90-105 dias — and always high the few times when taken at the surgery, (I'm pretty sure it isn't white coat syndrome) I knew that it was normal sometimes. So I started taking notes of its readings and what I was eating and doing. I'd sit quietly for 10 minutes before taking it.

In the last 4 years or so I had been on very low salt, which did nothing to help. I started eating more salt again, my BP came down, but went back up again after a few days.

I cut out added sugar. Similar result. I continue to eat very little added sugar.

I realise there are coincidences in eating that could also affect BP; at the same time I must have been eating or doing something else beneficial or otherwise, but then ceased. I think I eat good food, but there are a lot of possible details that can go unnoticed.

The Low Carb High Fat (LCHF) approach helped but maintaining it is the problem for me. It recommends animal protein, fat/oil, no added sugar and low carbs/starch. This means you eat very few starchy vegetables and grains/seeds.

If, like me, you like carbs such as bread, pasta and other similar things, LCHF is difficult to stick to. It creates cravings similar to those caused by low fat 'diets'. You can end up eating carbs anyway, and not in a good way.

Many of us like grain products but they can cause problems too. The staple diet of many cultures and countries is grains so we can't just reject them. But how are they traditionally eaten?

Whole grains contain protein, but are not the complete protein needed by humans. The addition of pulses (lentils, beans, peas, and the like) in their various forms completes the amino acids (protein) we need. I was taught that this then provides us with the same quality protein as animal products — meat, eggs, dairy, fish, etc. It is sometimes called Class 1 protein. Most pulses on their own also need grain to complete the amino acids.

Many cultures' traditional meals/foods include both grains and pulses, e.g. daal with pitta bread, fried rice and beans, meat with beans/lentils and rice, some Asian breads, beans on toast, peas and rice. Some grains and pulses such as quinoa and soya are complete protein on their own.

For me, the addition of the missing amino acids by combining grains and pulses in some foods, in particular form, and in conjunction with other (above) helpful alterations, instead of eating just wheat flour, brought my blood pressure down. By now I was eating a varied diet of animal protein, grain and pulse combination protein, adequate, generous fats/oil, fresh vegetables and fruit, a few starchy vegetables, some salt, and no added sugar, largely as meals. My BP was very good.

But then it went back up again.

I realise BP does go up and down during the day and have taken that into account. When good it goes up and down a bit at a good level. When high it goes up and down a bit at a high level.

I sometimes eat out and within reason always eat what is available or given to me. I have taken this into account. I don't think it matters on occasions as long as what I eat at home or regularly is within what I know to be good for my BP.

"Bread is the staff of life" is an archaic saying and to be true needs archaic bread. We don't really know what bread was made of originally but it certainly didn't have highly-processed flour in it. It would have been unleavened (flat bread) and have other things in it as well as grains.

Part of my eating during self experimenting was making a type of bread that included both grain and pulse (gram flour as pulse). It is a flat bread with spices and other ingredients in it and is of Indian origin. I ate it instead of usual wheat bread. I also made similar alterations to other food.

My BP was really good for a couple of weeks. However, after a while I found it was up again. But I think I now know what that was.

When making flat bread and other foods with grain flours and pulses, I had used wholemeal wheat flour. When I used it all up I later realised that I'd started using what was left — white flour — combined with pulses.

The benefits of wholemeal over white flour are commonly known. Wholemeal has the germ still in it and that is the most nutritious part of the grain. But because of this it doesn't keep as long as white flour. White flour has most of it removed, but that omission must mean the body can't then get some part of its protein or is missing some vital nutrient. And that it is then nutritionally diminished, whether combined with pulses or not.

This is why I think the ratio of protein to starch needs to be generous on the protein side — plus fats, of course. And we can help do that by eating the complete vegetable protein of combined whole grain/flour and pulses in particular ways.

White flour is largely starch. When eaten — with or without pulses — such as white bread, pasta etc., it may be treated by the body as mainly starch and at the very least just be converted to sugar by our bodies.

However, by providing that full protein our bodies deal with it or use it as such. But without the complimentary protein, we are eating higher sugar lower protein.

The main point of eating is to get protein and fats. Protein is used for building, repair and growth of our bodies and brains and nothing can substitute for it. (See earlier paragraph on protein and what our bodies need to be able to make full use of it.)

There is no way the body can store excess protein. It will be used as fuel instead. So eating grains and pulses at different times might not be optimum. It is said by some that as long as they are eaten within 24hours of each other then that is OK. However, most cultures' traditional ways of eating combine them in the same meal.

I am not diabetic so don't know what my blood sugar levels are. But possibly there is a cross-over in terms of starch converting to sugar, a large proportion of starch to protein, and elevated BP.

Having cut added sugar I don't miss it and now find many things too sweet.

I rarely eat potatoes and other starchy vegetables without protein, and then usually of animal origin, and then don't overdo their quantity. A few potatoes, or similar, roasted, fried, or boiled (butter or oil added), with decent protein and other vegetables, seem OK. An overload of them puts my BP up.

For the several months during my trials my BP had been really good. But in November it was high again. I was very disappointed. I looked through my notes and realised that as winter approached various seasonal evenings and celebrations had begun. I had been to several buffets that included sandwiches, pies, cakes, crisps, etc., and at home occasionally ate more in the way of starchy and sweet foods. So although I was aware of various foods putting my BP up, I had eaten them but thought I hadn't overdone it.

So back to the original way of low BP eating, and within about 24-36 hours it was low/normal again. However, it proved to me again that it is starch, largely in the form of various foods containing white flour, and added sugar that puts my BP up.

I had also got a bit carried away with adding salt again, on top of which a lot of party foods contain salt. I now think I had topped it up too much. Also, it is winter so I was not perspiring salt away, as in the summer.

Lots of people don't have high blood pressure. No-one really knows what anyone else eats. But there are common foods and ingredients out there of varying qualities and types which, by chance, can be included regularly or not, and in varying quantities. I am just adding my experiences to the mix. There are of course, other causes of high BP.

This approach to being able to eat carbs by completing the vegetable origin protein works for me. It leaves less residue starch. Finding more foods that really do it but don't overdo it, is on-going.

Since cutting starch and added sugar I have also found that my anxiety level has dropped. That awful feeling of panic at something, and you don't really know what, seems to have largely gone. Even things to worry about worry me less. Perhaps the stress to the body of not receiving the real food/nourishment necessary to build and heal translates to those feelings of anxiety.

I feel so much better for eating like this. My legs have stopped feeling weary, I don't feel sleepy all day. Now I generally feel very well and energetic. I was quite energetic before but it was always a bit of a battle. Now it is a pleasure.

It is March 2018 now. I started this experimental eating for lowering BP in August last year. Results have been consistent. My food trials continue. I will post anything on website.

Oct 2019

I have been eating high protein – largely of animal origin- and fats, and very low starch. To begin with I felt even better. But over the months I realised my energy and stamina dropped. I found however, that an intake of starch (not refined) helps. But not to the level of it being a regular, large, everyday intake. So for me, a moderately active person, some form of carbs and a little starch helps. But to keep my weight stable, along with using the appetite controls, a high protein and fats works over high starch and fats.

oOo

We all have times when we find we have more or less willpower over our eating. But willpower isn't something we either have or don't have; it is a matter of using the triggers we all have to activate appetite controls, providing us with what we think of as willpower; a smaller and more easily satisfied appetite.

Some people simply eat the right amount and stay at a stable, healthy weight. They don't have to exercise willpower; they just stop eating when they've had enough. Their Appetite Control System is being used. That's what we all need, and it is possible for every one of us to have it.